Longevity Training-Book2 –Define Your Purpose in Life

This book is a transcription and reproduction of the training course materials from Course #2 "What is your Purpose in Living?" from the Longevity Coaching Training Server.

Except for being printed instead of Audio/Visual, it is the same content presented in that course.

This second course and this book are designed to give you a full introduction into the second of the 10 Principles of Personal Longevity "Define Your Purpose in Life".

The second principle is all about the concept that if you plan to live a long time then you really need a solid purpose and goals to do so.

Without a will to live we will die early and will not enjoy what remaining life we do have. The objective of this Course #2 Book is to learn how to develop your own Life Purpose and Goals to help make a long life both more feasible and more enjoyable.

Longevity Training-Book2 –Define Your Purpose in Life

Copyright Page

The book is copyrighted for 2018

Longevity Training-Book 2-Define Your Purpose in Life

By Martin K. Ettington

ISBN: 9781729275016

Printed in the United States of America

Longevity Training-Book2 –Define Your Purpose in Life

Other books by Martin K. Ettington

Spiritual and Metaphysics Books:
Prophecy: A History and How to Guide
God Like Powers and Abilities
Enlightenment for Newbies
Removing Illusions to Find True
                Happiness
Using the Scientific Method to Study
                the Paranormal
A Compendium of Metaphysics and
                How to Guides (Six books
                together in one volume)
Love from the Heart
The Enlightenment Experience
Learn Your Soul's Purpose
Pursuing Enlightenment
A Modern Man's Search for Truth
Use Intuition and Prophecy to Improve
                Your Life
The Handbook of Spiritual and Energy
                Healing

Longevity & Immortality:
Physical Immortality: A History and
                How to Guide
The Commentaries of Living Immortals
Records of Extremely Long Lived
                Persons
Enlightenment and Immortality
Longevity Improvements from Science
The 10 Principles of Personal
                Longevity
Telomeres & Longevity
The Diets and Lifestyles of the Worlds
                Oldest Peoples
The Longevity Six Books Bundle

Science Fiction:
Out of This Universe
Personal Freedom-Parts 1 & 2
The Psychic Soldier Series:
     Book 1-Himalayan Journey
     Book 2-A Soldier is Born
     Book 3-Fighting For Right
     Book 4-Earth Protector
The Immortality Sci Fi Bundle

The God Like Powers Series:
Human Invisibility
Invulnerability and Shielding
Teleportation
Psychokinesis
Our Energy Body, Auras, and
Thoughtforms

The God Like Powers Series—
                Volume 1 Compilation
The Yoga Discovery Series:
Yoga-An Ancient Art Form
Hatha Yoga-Helping you Live Better
Raja Yoga-Through the Ages
The Yoga Discovery Package

Business & Coaching Books:
Creating, Paublishing, & Marketing
                Practitioner Ebooks
Building a Successful Longevity
                Coaching Business
Why Become a Coach?
The Professional Coaching Success
Trilogy
2020-Make Money Writing and Selling
                Books
The 2020 Handbook of High Paying
                Work Without a College Degree

Science, Technology, and Misc.
Future Predictions By and Engineer &
                Seer
The Unusual Science & Technology
                Bundle
The Real Atlantis-In the Eye of the
                Sahara
Are Cryptozoological Animals Real or
                Imaginary?
Real Time Travel Stories From a
                Psychic Engineer
Removing Limits On Our
                Consciousness-And
                Thinking Outside the Box
33 Incredible True Survival Stories
How to Survive Anything: From the
                Wilderness to Man Made
                Disasters
All About Mars Journeys and
                Settlement
Mining the Asteroid Belt

Ancient History
The Real Atlantis-In the Eye of the
Sahara
Ancient & Prehistoric Civilizations
Ancient & Prehistoric Civilizations-Book
                Two
The History of Antediluvian Giants
The Antediluvian History of Earth
Ancient Underground Cities and
                Tunnels
Strange Objects Which Should Not Exist

Longevity Training-Book2 –Define Your Purpose in Life

Strange and Ancient Places in the USA
A Theory of Ancient Prehistory And
    Giant Aliens
<u>Aliens and Space</u>
Aliens and Secret Technology
Aliens Are Already Among Us
Designing and Building Space Colonies
Humanity and the Universe

All About Moon Bases
All About Mars Journeys and Settlement
The Space and Aliens Six Books Bundle
A Theory of Ancient Prehistory and
    Giant Aliens
The Space Colonies and Space
    Structures Coloring Book
All About Asteroids

<u>The Longevity Training Series</u>

(A transcription of the online Multimedia Longevity Coaching Training Program)

The Personal Longevity Training Series-Book1-Long Lived Persons
The Personal Longevity Training Series-Book2-Your Soul's Purpose
The Personal Longevity Training Series-Book3-Enable Your Life Urge
The Personal Longevity Training Series-Book4-Your Spiritual Connection
The Personal Longevity Training Series-Book5-Having Love in Your Heart
The Personal Longevity Training Series-Book6-Energy Body Health
The Personal Longevity Training Series-Book7-The Science of Longevity
The Personal Longevity Training Series-Book8-Physical Body Health
The Personal Longevity Training Series-Book9-Avoiding Accidents
The Personal Longevity Training Series-Book10-Implementing These Principles

The Personal Longevity Training Series-Books One Thru Ten

These books are all available in digital and printed formats from my
website and on Amazon, Barnes & Noble, Apple ITunes, and many other sites

My Books Website is: http://mkettingtonbooks.com

Longevity Training-Book2 –Define Your Purpose in Life

<u>Signup for our Mailing List to get the following:</u>

1) A discount coupon for 25% discount on all books on our site

2) Occasional Notices of new books available

3) Occasional Email on other offerings of ours (Monthly)

Go to this link to sign-up:

http://personal-longevity.com/mkebooks/emailsignup/

And click this link to get the FREE 102 page Ebook titled "Secrets of Many Things"

If you have any questions about this book or other subjects please contact the Author at:

mke@mkettingtonbooks.com

Table of Contents

Longevity Training-Book2 –Define Your Purpose in Life

Introduction

Back in 2008 I became very interested in the field of Longevity and Physical Immortality. After a lot of research this led me to my first book on the subject "Physical Immortality: A History and How to Guide". This book was pretty popular and I wanted to continue learning about Longevity and what things we could do about it in our lives.

The subject continued to fascinate me to the point that I developed a Longevity Coaching program over a couple of years starting in 2011. This online training program was multimedia—consisting of videos, my writings on longevity to read, online exercises, and tests for each of ten courses. It also included a lot of additional resources for each course including extra courses on how to become a successful Longevity Coach. A student who completed the training and tests successfully would become certified as a "Longevity Coach" and authorized to teach this material to others.

I developed a set of ten principles on longevity which are as follows:

The 10 Principles of Personal Longevity are:

- The Reality of Long Lived People
- Defining Your Purpose in Life
- Enabling the Life Urge
- Your Spiritual Health
- Having Love in Your Heart
- Energy Body Health
- The Science of Longevity
- Physical Body Health
- Using your Intuition for Safety
- Implementation of these principles

What are the 10 Principles all about?

The Reality of Long Lived People

The first principle is where I provide lots of evidence of people who have lived well over the age of 120 years old to 150-180-200, and even a 256 year old man from China:

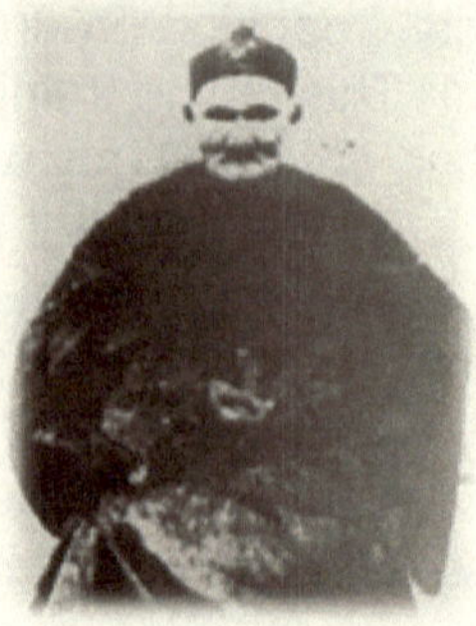

LI CHING-YUN: The Longest Lived person of record-256 Years (Source-The New York Times-May 6, 1933)

The Second Principle of Life Purpose

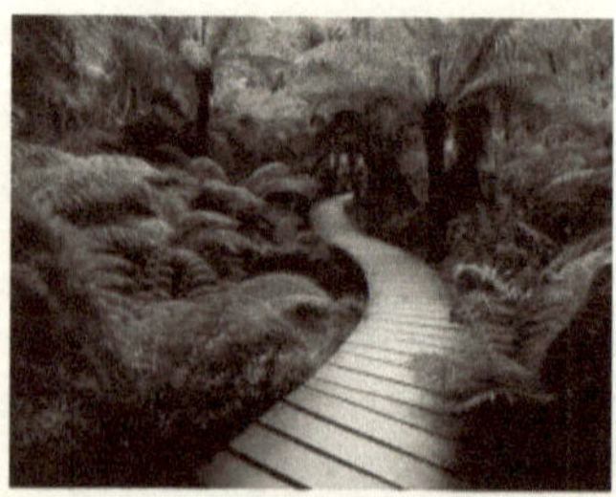

One of the things that occurred to me when I was putting the 10 principles together was that if one doesn't have a reason to live, or purpose in life--then what is the point?

This meant I had to add a very important step of how you can develop your own life purpose, or bring it up to date with your phase in life. Without reviewing your purpose-- then none of the rest of the principles matter.

Enabling the Life Urge

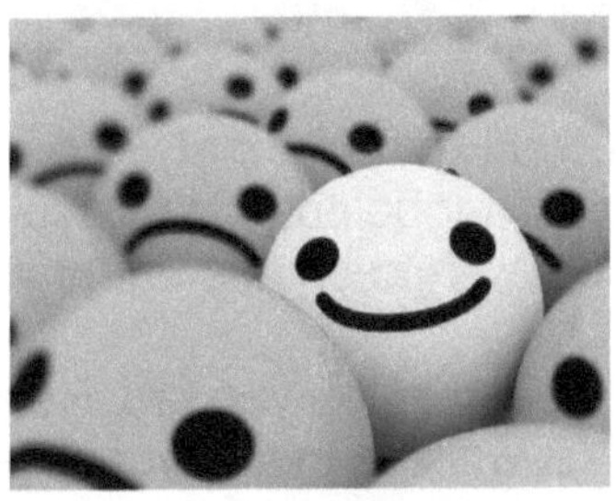

Have you ever realized how we are all programmed to expect to live through certain stages in life and then die? It's so common in our society that we don't think it odd that we expect to die at a certain age?

Have you ever heard radio ads saying "You are getting up in your sixties and seventies" so it's time to come out to our cemetery and buy a plot"

How ridiculous is this? And do you see how much our subconscious has been programmed towards death?

This principle is all about reprogramming ourselves to have a more positive outlook on life and its possibilities.

Having a Spiritual Connection in Your Life

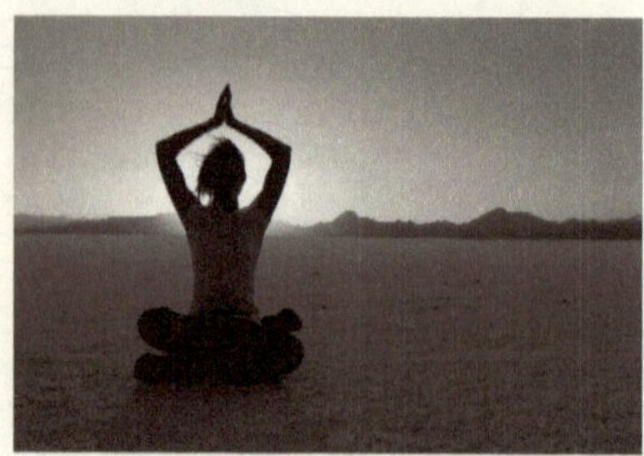

Most of us innately understand that we have a spiritual core in the center of our being. It is this spiritual core that we need to connect with to enable our physical health too.

It doesn't matter what religion you are. Regular meditation, deep prayer, or just walking in the woods helps you make and keep that connection in your life.

Having Love in Your Heart

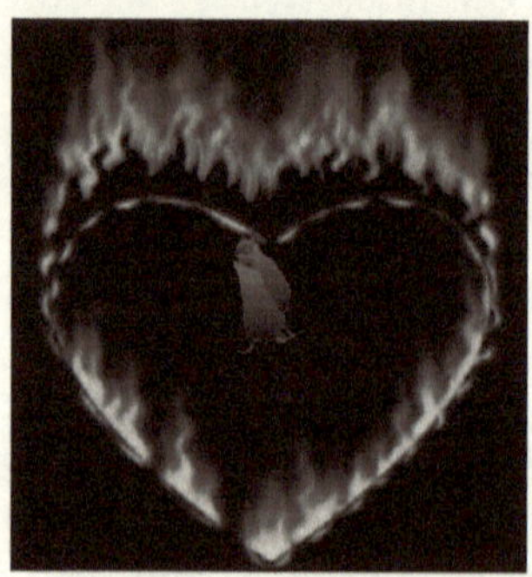

One of the most important things I learned in the last five years was that Unconditional Love is a real and physical thing. It is a powerful energy force in life and not just a philosophical belief system.

I considered it so important that I added it as a separate principle of longevity.

True Unconditional Love is healing, embodies happiness, and is a powerful part of our vital forces.

Energy Body Health

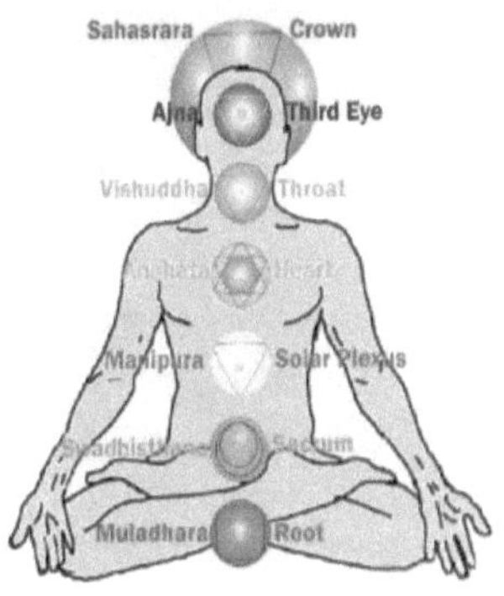

We all have an energy body which is part of our vital forces. The Indians talk about the "Chakras" and the Chinese talk about "Energy Meridians" in Acupuncture.

We should all learn different practices to keep our vital forces flowing for maximum health and vitality.

The Science of Longevity

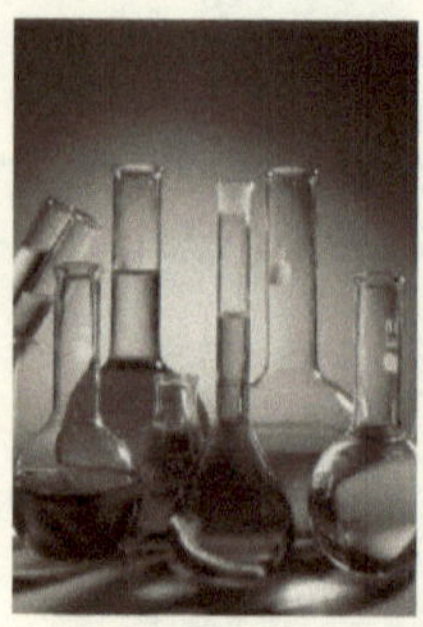

Science and Medicine are making new discoveries all the time that we can take advantage of to extend our lives. Why not take advantage of these discoveries which provide new therapies and supplements to increase our longevity.

There is also a lot we can learn from plants and animals. We all share the same genetic basis.

Some of these plants and animals live thousands of years and some cells are immortal.

What can we learn from them to apply to our lives?

Physical Body Health

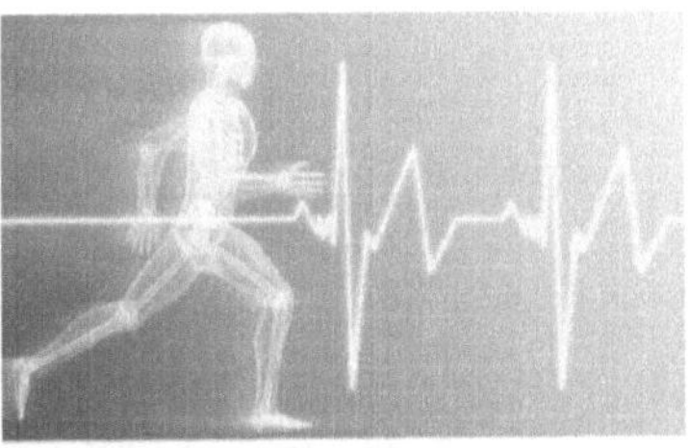

There are many types of supplements used for anti-aging for thousands of years. What can we learn about them that we can apply to our lives?

What other considerations about our physical health does nontraditional or alternative medicine offer?

Using Your Intuition for Safety

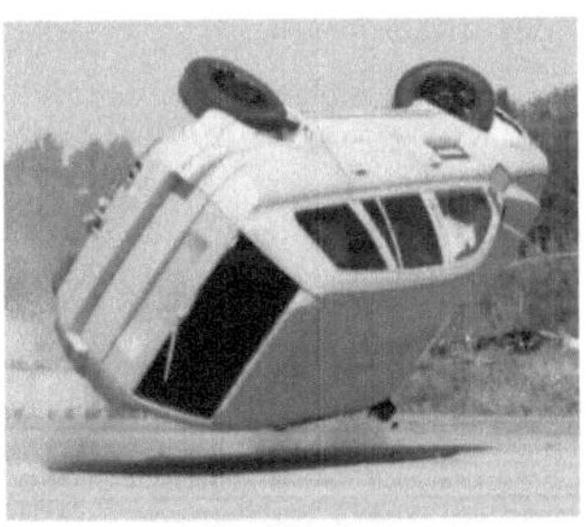

Once you have established your own long term health then what is the greatest danger you face?

ACCIDENTS

We can learn to use our intuition to make us safer as well as see potential future events which may be good too.

Why not open up to the possibilities of how our spirit has this natural ability in all of us?

Implementing These Principles in Your Life

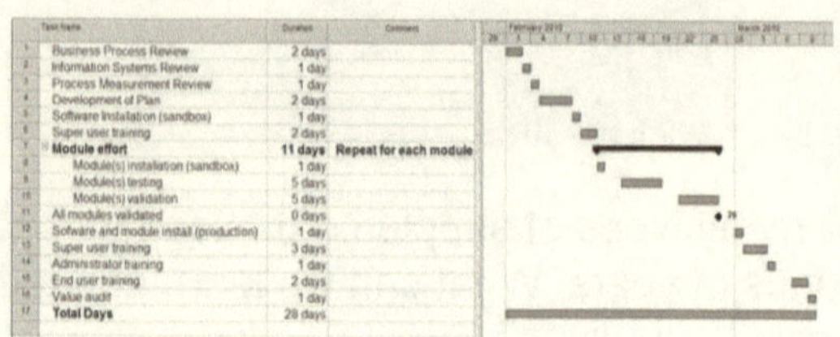

It's nice to read about all these concepts, but how can you really apply them to your own life?

This is what the chapter on implementation is all about, and it helps you plan a lifelong change in your health focus to live these principles and truly experience long term health, greater happiness, and extended longevity.

For five years I amended and improved these materials which now include a lot more information and helpful concepts for students wanting to improve their longevity and those of others.

I transcribed my videos and other materials to this book so you can read it all, and later hear it in an AudioBook.

This book is priced pretty inexpensively, compared to the online training and certification program which sells in total for $1,995 USD. If you are interested in taking the entire online program at a major discount, then please contact me at:

Marty@personal-longevity.com

Hope you enjoy these materials since when applied correctly they will significantly change your life.

PLP Concepts Overview

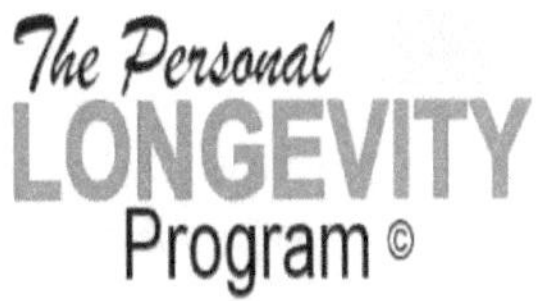

(Transcription of overview video)

Hello I'm Martin Ettington and I'd like to introduce you to the Personal Longevity Program which is an integrated holistic approach to long-term health. In this video we will only cover the high level concepts which comprise individual courses in the coaching certificate program for personal longevity.

The first concept is that long lived people exist and have existed for hundreds of thousands of years. We cover in the first course all about their records; along with people not only in places you might think like India, but in Europe and the United States-people who've lived long lives and well documented cases.

We discuss people who have lived well over the age of 120 and even the case of a Chinaman who lived to 256 years old. Plus a lot of mythology about people who have lived even longer lives so you get an idea that extending your life much longer than we think is currently medically and scientifically possible is certainly something that can happen.

The second course's concept has to do with finding your souls purpose. The point of wanting to live a long life is to know what your purpose in life is, so we go through some readings and some exercises to help you determine where soul's purpose in life is. Then doing goals as a fundamental concept so you will know the motivations in your life.

Third is the "Psychology of Living" also known by certain practitioners as "Removing the death Urge". The psychology of living has to do with seeking a positive image about your ability to live a long time. We tend to be programmed from birth about the idea that we are going to go through certain stages in our life as a child, as a teenager, and as adults. It's about reprogramming your subconscious as to the possibilities of a long life.

I've also learned in my life that it is very important to be able open your heart to unconditional love. When you're able to love unconditionally it also helps increase the strength of your immune system and fight off disease. So this is an aspect of spiritual growth. The courses also cover unconditional love and energy body forces. Managing your energy body is an important component of who you are in having energy working properly in your body and is another aspect of health for the length of longevity.

There are many types of scientific and medical research which are being done today and which will contribute to human longevity in the future.

Do you know that the average lifespan in the United States in 1900 was only about 40 years? We have doubled lifespan in the last century with current technologies but things under way in terms of scientific and medical improvements will help extend your lives further.

Also in this course on longevity we will cover a lot of the concepts which are being researched by scientists today. There are suggestions for more things you can do to do to use this science to improve your health along with physical supplements.

A unique thing that I thought about and decided to offer in these courses has to do with all my experiences in prophecy and how I was able to change outcomes on accidents that would occur to me by using simple exercises you can learn to change these outcomes. If you're in great health often the biggest thing you have to worry about are accidents.

We also provide guidelines you can follow on a daily basis and plans you can make to live healthier and happier and have a much longer life than you ever thought possible.

Thank you for listening !

Longevity Training-Book2 –Define Your Purpose in Life

Course #2 Introduction Video

(Video Transcription)

Hello-This is Marty Ettington and I'd like to welcome you to Course Number Two of the Personal Longevity Program on "What is Your Purpose in Living".

One of the things that I was thinking about when I put this entire sequence of 10 courses together was why would people want to live and extended life? That if you don't have a real purpose in life or reason to be on this earth and what's the point… all the rest of it doesn't really matter.

So I read a lot of material, I consult a lot of friends; there's a lot of life purpose coaches out there these days-I talk to them…. and I came up with this course which I think is a key element of the longevity process.

You really have to know your life purpose if you want to be happy and successful and fulfilled in your lifetime. So let's get into what we cover in this course.

First of all it's important to think of what life is like without a purpose. And what that really means is that if there is no meaning in your life you float around and let random events determine what you going to do. And again, it doesn't really provide you with a reason to want to live a long time.

So this reinforces the importance of finding your Soul's purpose. And what would I call that? To live a life in the flow of your spirit with maximum happiness and satisfaction. And if you were her life's purpose or your sole purpose and you really try to follow it you can do that. So part of this is how their spiritual connection relates to purpose. Because we all have part of the eternal spirit at the core of our being.

A lot of writers and a lot of our people in this business believe that if you're not connected to your spirit, to determine where sole purpose is you will not know what it is, you will not find and therefore you'll be drifting-or you will relieve you of really be happy with what you're doing. So building a spiritual connection is important, and that's one of the Assignments having to do that.

Another area is on hoping to write a life purpose or Soul purpose statement. And this is based on information from a book, which is very good called "Becoming a Professional Life Coach" By Patrick Williams and Diane Menendez. And they have a great section which I took for this exercise on going through with a different stages to write a life purpose for Soul purpose statement-from which you can then develop specific goals.

Also, another aspect which is important has to do with the power of your thought.

There is an old classic over 100 years old, called "The Science of Getting Rich" which you might not think it is applicable to this, but it really has to do with a big focus on the power of your thinking; both subconsciously and consciously to meeting your goals. So once you develop your life purpose statement and your goals-having some control of your thoughts and focus will help you manifest what you really want to do.

So some other resources in this course have to do with another book I wrote: "Your Soul's Purpose to Live a Fulfilling Life". Additional purpose Ebooks "The Science of Getting Rich" And then in the Additional Resources Page which is the last assignment link you can look at different Law of Attraction books and some other links to purpose books on my website MKEttingtonBooks.com

So I hope you enjoy the course and don't forget to do the test at the end which is certainly important especially if you want to get the certificates for the full series of 10 courses

Thank You.

Your Soul's Purpose

(Selected Chapters from the Book "Learn Your Soul's Purpose")

Introduction

The reason I decided to write this book was because I was putting together a sequence of courses towards a certificate program in Health and Longevity.

One of the things I soon realized was that without an individual's will to live, they will never desire or make the effort to live a long and fulfilling life.

Therefore, each of us has to have developed a fundamental purpose in life-to live life to the fullest.

Without that purpose there is no meaning in what we do.

The goal of this book is therefore to help you do introspection as to whether you have a well-developed life purpose.

If you do know your life purpose—then congratulations!

If not—then I hope these lessons will lead you towards better understanding your purpose in life.

Life Without a Purpose

The Dalai Lama sums up the lack of purpose in many of our lives today:

> *We have more conveniences, but less time.*

> *We have more degrees, but less sense more knowledge but less judgment. More experts, but more problems. More medicines, but less healthiness.*

> *We have been all the way to the moon and back but have trouble crossing the street to meet the new neighbor.*

> *We build more computers to hold more information that produce more copies than ever before, but have less communication.*

> *We have become long on quantity, but short on quality. These are the times of fast foods but weak digestion. It is a time when there is much in the window but nothing in the room.*

Not knowing one's purpose is one of the biggest problems in life around the world today.

Not everyone can be a gifted composer or scientist—yet we all have a true uniqueness as our gift from God.

Each of us has at least one unique thing to contribute to this world-ourselves.

Maybe your purpose in life it to be a friend to others, or to just provide some comfort to a person in need.

Our life purpose doesn't have to be big—it just has to be something from deep in our Soul that satisfies our reason for incarnating in this life.

How I know my Soul's Purpose

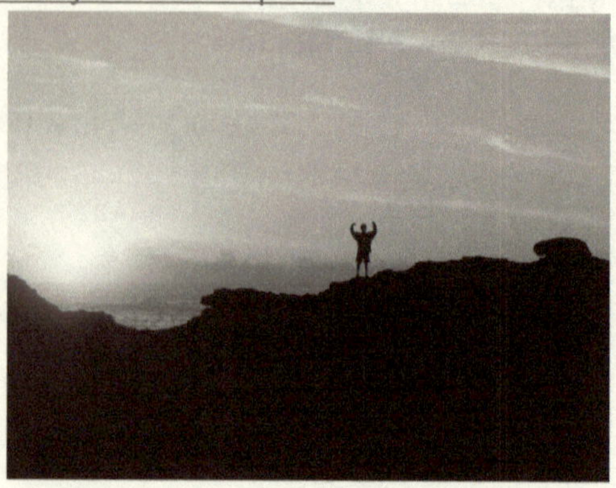

I have been blessed with many wonderful experiences in my life.

The first blessing in my life was that I remember before I was born, my gestation, and my birth.

I remember being part of a larger super consciousness in another realm of the spirit. That I felt the need to return to the earth to accomplish a new mission.

Other similar consciousnesses around me told me that I had already done a lot of work on the earth and didn't need to go back. My decision was firm though—I knew this incarnation needed to be accomplished and I was determined to do it.

I broke off a portion of my spirit into a smaller package and came down to the earth to choose a mother and father.

My recollection is that my goal in choosing parents was to find a pair of well-educated parents who would be well grounded in life-thus raising me to be well grounded.

There were several candidate couples in upstate New York. I choose a candidate and came closer to my new mother to be. When I got close I was drawn inside of her womb and my spirit became attached to the embryo growing there.

At one point the cord was choking me so I had to turn around to get it from around my neck.

I remember growing in my mom's womb—then it became too small and I felt compressed. Eventually it became so tight that my mom's water broke and I started being forced out.

I was a breach birth and came out feet first. The compression pain was great when I passed through my mom's birth canal/

After I was born I recall breathing on my own. Then the doctor held me up and hit my butt—I spasmed and took in a great breath of air—which felt like fire in my lungs. His overly powerful slap of my bottom also caused congestion in my lungs so I was placed in an iron lung for a few hours.

 At the age of two years old I was sitting in my living room watching an old boxy black and white TV—then I remember that I was waking up from some type of dream I'd been living for the last couple of years. That I knew I was alive and here to accomplish my mission on earth!

Much of my teenage years were consumed with curiosity about the spiritual and paranormal. Without much information available from my parents and friends I found books to read which satisfied my thirst for knowledge.

Throughout my childhood I still knew that I had an important purpose in life—but wasn't sure what it was.

Later in my teens I was drawn to read books on the paranormal, try ESP experiments read lots of Science Fiction.

In college I met a spiritual Mentor named Sam Lentine who taught me how to meditate, and to take in energy through my crown chakra.

In parallel with a traditional business career for thirty years, I had many spiritual and paranormal experiences. (Which I've covered in some of my other books)

In 2008 I just felt it was time to start writing on what I could research and what I knew about different spiritual and paranormal subjects.

Now in early 2013 I know that the last four years I was building a foundation of knowledge, books, videos, and other materials to prepare me for my real life's work..

My real life's work turns out to be that of a Spiritual Teacher and counselor on long term health and extreme longevity.

How do I know this? It's not an analytical answer but a spiritual one—that now I feel I'm in spiritual alignment with my life's purpose.

This alignment makes me excited about the future, and I can't wait to implement my training program.

My alignment with my spirit's goals energizes me and just gives me a deep "knowing" that I'm on the right track.

It's hard to express, but I just know I was meant to be on this path.

Everything I've learned and experienced up until this point in life is part of this path.

My point in relating the above story was to show how I became certain of my life's purpose. Hopefully you will have a similar awakening.

Having these types of feelings about your life is how you know you have found your life's calling.

You don't need to go through all of the events of my life to find your Soul's Purpose.

By introspection and some of the exercises offered later in this book you can find what that purpose really is.

Who you Really are

A good starting point on defining your Soul's Purpose is to determine who you really are. You should ask questions of your family and friends to help you better grasp why you are here:

- What are you reflecting back to yourself by not allowing yourself to see or know your Soul's purpose?

- Who supports you in living your Soul's purpose and who does not support you?

- Who of all of your friends would be there for you to support you in discovering your Soul's purpose and following through with you on bringing it to the surface?

- Ask each family member, young or old; what do they think is your Soul's purpose?

Write down each person's answer, without comment or judgment. Also, ask each personal friend or co-worker what they think is your Soul's purpose. This will help you in discovering your Soul's purpose.

> *Once you realize what your Soul's purpose is – you will stop wasting your time by distracting yourself from what you really aught to be doing.-Deborah Skye King*

Many cases of depression and listlessness are the result of not knowing what you are meant to do on this earth in this lifetime.

The joy and happiness you experience in life are in many ways linked to how well you are working towards your life's path or purpose.

Did you ever see a depressed person who was doing their real life's work? Or a person energized about their work if they saw no purpose to it?

Your Mission in Life

Why is it important to have a mission in life? Here are some quotes from the Bible that may help answer that question:

> It is God himself who has made us what we are and given us new lives from Christ Jesus; and long ages ago he planned that we should spend these lives in helping others. Ephesians 2:10

> I glorified you on earth by completing down to the last detail what you assigned me to do. John 17:4

You were put on earth to make a contribution.

You weren't created just to consume resources—to eat, breathe, and take up space. God designed you to make a difference with your life. While many best-selling books offer advice on how to "get" the most out of life, that's not the reason God made you. You were created to add to life on earth, not just take from it. God wants you to give something back. This is God's fourth purpose for your life, and it is called your "ministry," or service. The Bible gives us the details. You were created to serve God.

- The Purpose Driven Life: What on Earth Am I Here For? By Rick Warren

Building a Life Purpose

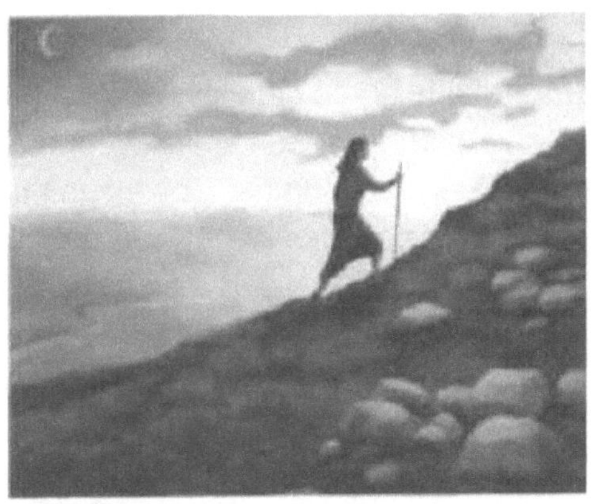

What is Purpose?

Ancient writers wrote a lot about this topic. An ancient Tibetan text states that a life purpose is *"for the benefit of self and for the benefit of others."*

Below are four quotations relevant to the issue of life purpose that we give to ILCT participants, asking them to reflect on what the quotes mean to them. These four seem to be particularly meaningful quotations that move students toward introspective thinking about the importance of life purpose and the variety of ways to describe it.

- When we are motivated by goals that have deep meaning, by dreams that need completion, by pure love that needs expressing, then we truly live life.

- We can define "purpose" in several ways. For one, when we know our purpose, we have an anchor— a device of the mind to provide some stability, to keep from tossing us to and fro, from inflicting constant seasickness on us. Or we can think of our purpose as being a master nautical chart marking shoals and rocks, sandbars and derelicts, something to guide us and keep us on course. Perhaps the most profound thing we can say about being "on purpose" is that when that is our status, our condition, and our comfort, we find our lives have meaning, and when we are "off purpose," we are confused about meanings and motives.

- The first principle of ethical power is Purpose. . . . By purpose, I mean your objective or intention— something toward which you are always striving. Purpose is something bigger. It is the picture you have of yourself— the kind of person you want to be or the kind of life you want to lead.

- A purpose is more ongoing and gives meaning to our lives. . . . When people have a purpose in life, they enjoy everything they do more! People go on chasing goals to prove something that doesn't have to be proved: that they're already worthwhile.

There are a variety of techniques we can use to zero in on our true life purpose.

Here are some exercises to help you create a life purpose statement:

(From Becoming a Professional Life Coach)

1. List the top ten things you love to do or have always done and loved. Name several things you have consistently made part of your life, regardless of the circumstances. Examples might include networking with like-minded people, your faith or spirituality, your creativity at work, your heartfelt communications, or your ability to take action under pressure.

2. Identify the characteristics of the context or environment that support your list from Step 1. List the qualities of people you want and need to be around to accomplish your top ten. Draw a series of concentric circles on a blank piece of paper, and write "ME" in the center circle. Each circle represents a group of people who are important to you. Put the names of those closest to you, who affect your life most, in the circle next to you. Then continue to draw your circles outward: family, friends, work colleagues, professional groups, community, and so on. In each circle, write a few words that describe the qualities this group must embody to support you in just the way you need and want. Then identify other resources that are essential to you: peacefulness, time in nature, other creative people, and so on. Ask yourself, "What are the essential supporting

features of the world I want to live in so that I can be at my best?"

3. Using the phrases you generated in Step 2, write one to two sentences that express your vision of the world you want to live in. This is the path of least resistance for you, the world you flourish in and want to create for yourself through purpose-full action. Crystallize the essence of your vision. For example, "My vision is that all people of the world will be able to live their lives by choice— in a way that matters to them." This vision expresses the fact that choice is essential for the writer.

Once we have a long term purpose then extended longevity (physical immortality) becomes an important goal to strive for.

Setting Goals

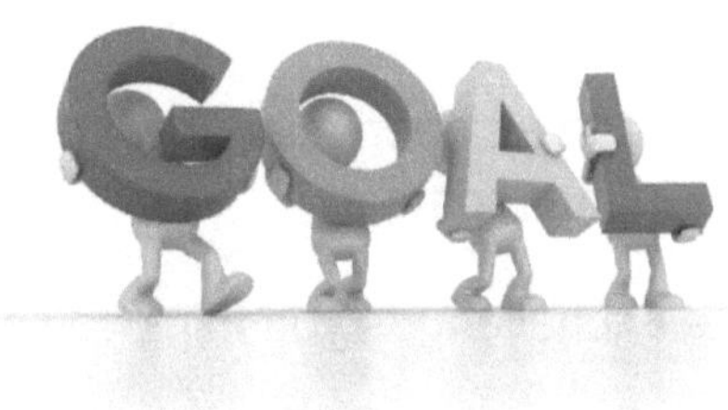

Once you have developed your life purpose it's time to set goals to accomplish it.

Only 3% of the world's population set goals—and they accomplish more than the other 97% combined.

Dr. John F. Dimartini describes the process of goal setting:

- Goals are to be of a realistic nature.

- Goals are to be believable to you and achievable.

- Goals are to be specific, the more detail the better.

- Goals are to be harmonious with your higher values. They should be created with what you already know or are interested in.

- Goals are to be prioritized; having a list of what you desire creates a stronger foundation from which to work.

- Goals are to be given completion and achievement dates. This way you can have markers for what is being created and what you need to do in order to complete a goal.

Setting a Course of Action:

1) Begin the day with an open mind toward what you desire to create in the moment

2) Write down any challenges you think you may encounter

3) Set up a plan for how you will accomplish your goals

4) If any challenges occur, remember to have a marker, something that will show you that you have arrived at your predetermined destination, so you will know you have accomplished what you have set out to.

Living in Awareness

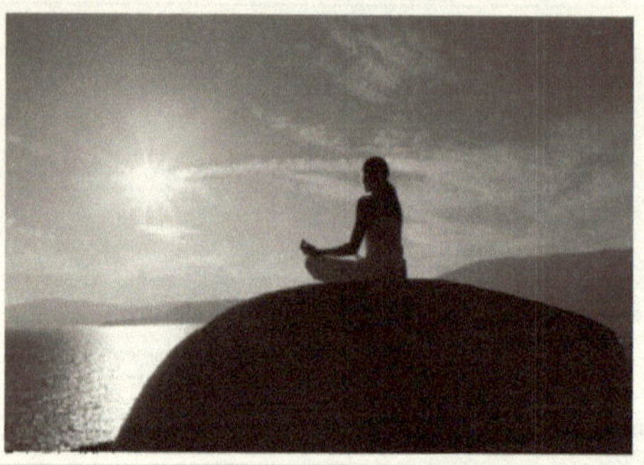

We should learn to bring awareness from the Soul to everything we do.

This allows us to be authentic—to know our real selves.

When we do this we are more in touch with our Soul's needs and purpose in life.

Do you give thanks for everything you do?

How about when you are brushing your teeth in the morning—do you give thanks for that action?

Do you notice the pleasure you have in each bite of food you take?

Do you think about the words you are saying to others and their effect on them and you?

What about thanks for your every breath—without continuous breathing you wouldn't last very long.

Living in awareness is all about clearly seeing and experiencing our environment from minute to minute—and living in the present.

Being aware at this level helps you to understand if you are doing something worthwhile or living in emptiness.

This level of awareness will also help you live in the heart to experience unconditional love too.

Longevity Training-Book2 –Define Your Purpose in Life

Alternatives Analysis Video

This video shows a spreadsheet which is used to help the student analyze alternatives for any set of goals or alternative opportunities.

(Video Transcription)

Hello. In this lesson we're going to do some alternatives analysis of the goals or alternatives that you came up with as part of the Soul purpose exercise.

What you will need for this is either in a spreadsheet you can use a computer or a printed form to do this manually.

This is a great technique which I've used in business for many years and there's no reason we can't apply it to the Soul Purpose exercises.

So what you are going to do is to open the PDF file in this assignment to see the instructions on how the spreadsheet works and then download the spreadsheet yourself and put in your alternatives you want to measure, ranking criteria and go ahead and see how it works out for you.

I'd like to see that spreadsheet uploaded to the question in the test so you I can see how did. Okay –Good Luck!

(See next page for a snapshot of the alternatives spreadsheet)

The following callout boxes point to the spreadsheet:

- Put your evaluation criteria which are important to you here
- Rank your criteria by importance here
- Put in your raw scores as to how this choice ranks on eval criteria here
- The spreadsheet calculates weighted totals here
- The weighted totals or scores for each alternative are in blue and you can see that this one is the best alternative based on ranking and weighting criteria

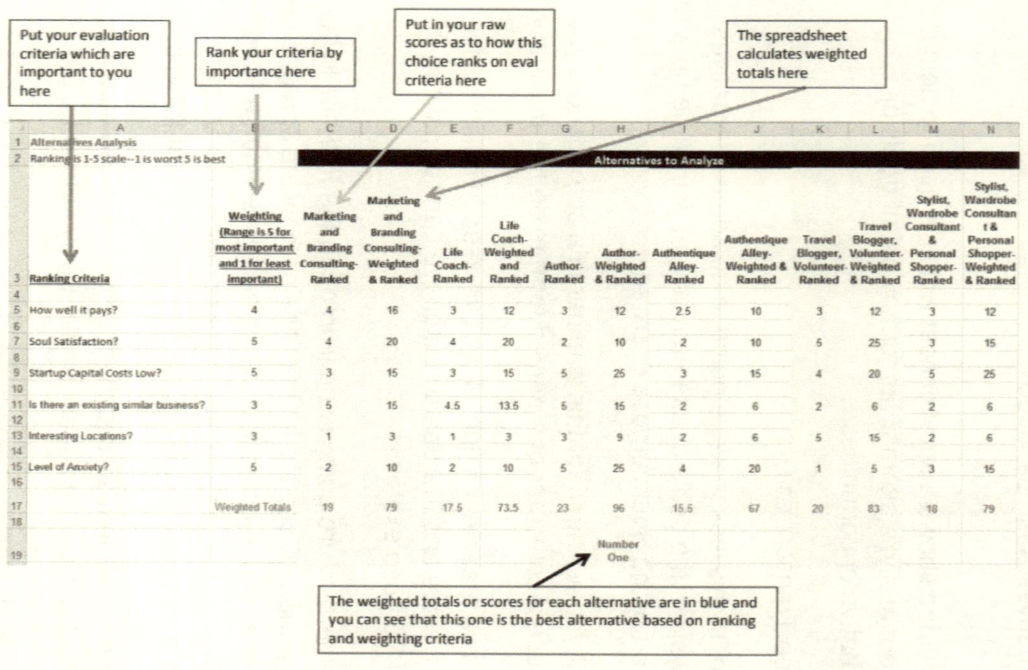

	A	B	C	D	E	F	G	H	I	J	K	L	M	N
1	Alternatives Analysis													
2	Ranking is 1-5 scale--1 is worst 5 is best						Alternatives to Analyze							
3	Ranking Criteria	Weighting (Range is 5 for most important and 1 for least important)	Marketing and Branding Consulting- Ranked	Marketing and Branding Consulting- Weighted & Ranked	Life Coach- Ranked	Life Coach- Weighted and Ranked	Author- Ranked	Author- Weighted & Ranked	Authentique Alley- Ranked	Authentique Alley- Weighted & Ranked	Travel Blogger, Volunteer- Ranked	Travel Blogger, Volunteer- Weighted & Ranked	Stylist, Wardrobe Consultant & Personal Shopper- Ranked	Stylist, Wardrobe Consultant & Personal Shopper- Weighted & Ranked
5	How well it pays?	4	4	16	3	12	3	12	2.5	10	3	12	3	12
7	Soul Satisfaction?	5	4	20	4	20	2	10	2	10	5	25	3	15
9	Startup Capital Costs Low?	5	3	15	3	15	5	25	3	15	4	20	5	25
11	Is there an existing similar business?	3	5	15	4.5	13.5	5	15	2	6	2	6	2	6
13	Interesting Locations?	3	1	3	1	3	3	9	2	6	5	15	2	6
15	Level of Anxiety?	5	2	10	2	10	5	25	4	20	1	5	3	15
17		Weighted Totals	19	79	17.5	73.5	23	96	15.5	67	20	83	18	79
19								Number One						

The Science of Getting Well—Chapters 1,4, 6

The below book is titled "The Science of Getting Well" By Wallace D Wattles. It is a classic text which is over 100 years old. The point of reading chapters 1, 4, and 6 is to see the way the author expresses his beliefs about the power of thought and visualization to reaching your goals.

The whole book is great but for brevity in the assignment I've picked these chapters:

Chapter 1-The Principle of Health

Chapter 4-What to think

Chapter 6-The Use of the Will

Many books and videos have been done on this subject in recent years, but these truths abide--that if you know what you really want, and can visualize the result properly, then you will achieve the goals.

Reason for this assignment: To review the power of thought and visualization to achieve your goals.

Benefits to Students: New techniques and reinforcement of approaches to help you achieve your goals. If you keep this mindset--it will happen.

Chapter 1

CHAPTER I. 5 CHAPTER II. THE FOUNDATIONS OF FAITH. Before man can think in the Certain Way which will cause his diseases to be healed, he must believe in certain truths which are here stated:-- All things are made from one Living Substance, which, in its original state, permeates, penetrates, and fills the interspaces of the universe. While all visible things are made from It, yet this Substance, in its first formless condition is in and through all the visible forms that It has made. Its life is in All, and its intelligence is in All. This Substance creates by thought, and its method is by taking the form of that which it thinks about. The thought of a form held by this substance causes it to assume that form; the thought of a motion causes it to institute that motion. Forms are created by this substance in moving itself into certain attitudes or positions. When Original Substance wishes to create a given form, it thinks of the motions which will produce that form. When it wishes to create a world, it thinks of the motions, perhaps extending through ages, which will result in its coming into the attitude and form of the world; and these motions are made. When it wishes to create an oak tree, it thinks of the sequences of movement, perhaps extending through ages, which will result in the form of an oak tree; and these motions are made. The particular sequences of motion by which differing forms should be produced were established in the beginning; they are changeless. Certain motions instituted in the Formless Substance will forever produce certain forms. Man's body is formed from the Original Substance, and is the result of certain motions, which first existed as thoughts of Original Substance. The motions which produce, renew, and repair the body of man are called functions, and these functions are of two classes: voluntary and involuntary. The involuntary functions are under the control of the Principle of Health in man, and are performed in a perfectly healthy manner so long as man thinks in a certain way. The voluntary functions of life are eating, drinking, breathing, and sleeping. These, entirely or in part, are under the direction of man's conscious mind; and he can perform them in a perfectly healthy way if he will. If he does not perform them in a healthy way, he cannot long be well. So we see that if man thinks in a certain way, and eats, drinks, breathes, and sleeps in a corresponding way, he will be well. The involuntary functions of man's life are under the direct control of the Principle of Health, and so long as man thinks in a perfectly healthy way, these functions are perfectly performed; for the action of the Principle of Health is largely directed by man's conscious thought, affecting his sub-conscious mind. Man is a thinking center, capable of originating thought; and as he does not know everything, he makes mistakes and thinks error. Not knowing everything, he believes things to be true which are not true. Man holds in his thought the idea of diseased and abnormal functioning and conditions, and so perverts the action of the Principle of Health, causing diseased and abnormal functioning and conditions within his own body. In the Original Substance there are held only the thoughts of perfect motion; perfect and healthy function; complete life. God never thinks disease or imperfection. But for countless ages men have held thoughts of disease, abnormality, old age, and death; and the perverted functioning resulting from these thoughts has become a part of the inheritance of the race. Our ancestors have, for many generations, held imperfect ideas concerning human form and functioning; and we begin life with racial sub-conscious impressions of imperfection and disease. This is not natural, or a part of the plan of nature. The purpose of nature can be nothing else than the perfection of life. This we see from the very nature of life itself. It is the nature of life to continually advance toward more perfect living; advancement is the inevitable result of the very act of living. Increase is always the result of active living; whatever lives must live more and more. The seed, lying in the granary, has life, but it is not living. Put it into the soil and it becomes active, and at once begins to gather to itself from the surrounding substance, and to build a plant form.

Chapter 4

CHAPTER IV. WHAT TO THINK. In order to sever all mental relations with disease, you must enter into mental relations with health, making the process positive not negative; one of assumption, not of rejection. You are to receive or appropriate health rather than to reject and deny disease. Denying disease accomplishes next to nothing; it does little good to cast out the devil and leave the house vacant, for he will presently return with others worse than himself. When you enter into full and constant mental relations with health, you must of necessity cease all relationship with disease. The first step in the Science of Being Well is, then, to enter into complete thought connection with health. The best way to do this is to form a mental image or picture of yourself as being well, imagining a perfectly strong and healthy body; and to spend sufficient time in contemplating this image to make it your habitual thought of yourself. This is not so easy as it sounds; it necessitates the taking of considerable time for meditation, and not all persons have the imaging faculty well enough developed to form a distinct mental picture of themselves in a perfect or idealized body. It is much easier, as in "The Science of Getting Rich," to form a mental image of the things one wants to have; for we have seen these things, or their counterparts, and know how they look; we can picture them very easily from memory. But we have never seen ourselves in a perfect body, and a clear mental image is hard to form. It is not necessary or essential, however, to have a clear mental image of yourself as you wish to be; it is only essential to form a

CONCEPTION of perfect health, and to relate yourself to it. This Conception of Health is not a mental picture of a particular thing; it is an understanding of health, and carries with it the idea of perfect functioning in every part and organ. You may TRY to picture yourself as perfect in physique; that helps; and you MUST think of yourself as doing everything in the manner of a perfectly strong and healthy person. You can picture yourself as walking down the street with an erect body and a vigorous stride; you can picture yourself as doing your day's work easily and with surplus vigor, never tired or weak; you can picture in your mind how all things would be done by a person full of health and power, and you can make yourself the central figure in the picture, doing things in just that way. Never think of the ways in which weak or sickly people do things; always think of the way strong people do things. Spend your leisure time in thinking about the Strong Way, until you have a good conception of it; and always think of yourself in connection with the Strong Way of Doing Things. That is what I mean by having a Conception of Health. In order to establish perfect functioning in every part, man does not have to study anatomy or physiology, so that he can form a mental image of each separate organ and address himself to it. He does not have to "treat" his liver, his kidneys, his stomach, or his heart. There is one Principle of Health in man, which has control over all the involuntary functions of his life; and the thought of perfect health, impressed upon this Principle, will reach each part and organ. Man's liver is not controlled by a liver-principle, his stomach by a digestive principle, and so on; the Principle of Health is One. The less you go into the detailed study of physiology, the better for you. Our knowledge of this science is very imperfect, and leads to imperfect thought. Imperfect thought causes imperfect functioning, which is disease. Let me illustrate: Until quite recently, physiology fixed ten days as the extreme limit of man's endurance without food; it was considered that only in exceptional cases could he survive a longer fast. So the impression became universally disseminated that one who was deprived of food must die in from five to ten days; and numbers of people, when cut off from food by shipwreck, accident, or famine, did die within this period. But the performances of Dr. Tanner, the forty-day faster, and the writings of Dr. Dewey and others on the fasting cure, together with the experiments of numberless people who have fasted from forty to sixty days, have shown that man's ability to live without food is vastly greater than had been supposed. Any person, properly educated, can fast from twenty to forty days with little loss in weight, and often with no apparent loss of strength at all. The people who starved to death in ten days or less did so because they believed that death was inevitable; an erroneous physiology had given them a wrong thought about themselves. When a man is deprived of food he will die in from ten to fifty days, according to the way he has been taught; or, in other words, according to the way he thinks about it. So you see that an erroneous physiology can work very mischievous results. No Science of Being Well can be founded on current physiology; it is not sufficiently exact in its knowledge. With all its pretensions, comparatively little is really known as to the interior workings and processes of the body. It is not known just how food is digested; it is not known just what part food plays, if any, in the generation of force. It is not known exactly what the liver, spleen, and pancreas are for, or what part their secretions play in the chemistry of assimilation. On all these and most other points we theorize, but we do not really know. When man begins to study physiology, he enters the domain of theory and disputation; he comes among conflicting opinions, and he is bound to form mistaken ideas concerning himself. These mistaken ideas lead to the thinking of wrong thoughts, and this leads to perverted functioning and disease. All that the most perfect knowledge of physiology could do for man would be to enable him to think only thoughts of perfect health, and to eat, drink, breathe, and sleep in a perfectly healthy way; and this, as we shall show, he can do without studying physiology at all. This, for the most part, is true of all hygiene. There are certain fundamental propositions which we should know; and these will be explained in later chapters, but aside from these propositions, ignore physiology and hygiene. They tend to fill your mind with thoughts of imperfect conditions, and these thoughts will produce the imperfect conditions in your own body. You cannot study any "science" which recognizes disease, if you are to think nothing but health. Drop all investigation as to your present condition, its causes, or possible results, and set yourself to the work of forming a conception of health. Think about health and the possibilities of health; of the work that may be done and the pleasures that may be enjoyed in a condition of perfect health. Then make this conception your guide in thinking of yourself; refuse to entertain for an instant any thought of yourself which is not in harmony with it. When any idea of disease or imperfect functioning enters your mind, cast it out instantly by calling up a thought which is in harmony with the Conception of

Health. Think of yourself at all times as realizing conception; as being a strong and perfectly healthy personage; and do not harbor a contrary thought. KNOW that as you think of yourself in unity with this conception, the Original Substance which permeates and fills the tissues of your body is taking form according to the thought; and know that this Intelligent Substance or mind stuff will cause function to be performed in such a way that your body will be rebuilt with perfectly healthy cells. The Intelligent Substance, from which all things are made, permeates and penetrates all things; and so it is in and through your body. It moves according to its thoughts; and so if you hold only the thoughts of perfectly healthy function, it will cause the movements of perfectly healthy function within you. Hold with persistence to the thought of perfect health in relation to yourself; do not permit yourself to think in any other way. Hold this thought with perfect faith that it is the fact, the truth. It is the truth so far as your mental body is concerned. You have a mind-body and a physical body; the mind-body takes form just as you think of yourself, and any thought which you hold continuously is made visible by the transformation of the physical body into its image. Implanting the thought of perfect functioning in the mind-body will, in due time, cause perfect functioning in the physical body. The transformation of the physical body into the image of the ideal held by the mind-body is not accomplished instantaneously; we cannot transfigure our physical bodies at will as Jesus did. In the creation and recreation of forms, Substance moves along the fixed lines of growth it has established; and the impression upon it of the health thought causes the healthy body to be built cell by cell. Holding only thoughts of perfect health will ultimately cause perfect functioning; and perfect functioning will in due time produce a perfectly healthy body. It may be as well to condense this chapter into a syllabus:-- Your physical body is permeated and fitted with an Intelligent Substance, which forms a body of mind-stuff. This mind-stuff controls the functioning of your physical body. A thought of disease or of imperfect function, impressed upon the mind-stuff, causes disease or imperfect functioning in the physical body. If you are diseased, it is because wrong thoughts have made impressions on this mind-stuff; these may have been either your own thoughts or those of your parents; we begin life with many sub-conscious impressions, both right and wrong. But the natural tendency of all mind is toward health, and if no thoughts are held in the conscious mind save those of health, all internal functioning will come to be performed in a perfectly healthy manner. The Power of Nature within you is sufficient to overcome all hereditary impressions, and if you will learn to control your thoughts, so that you shall think only those of health, and if you will perform the voluntary functions of life in a perfectly healthy way, you can certainly be well.

Chapter 6

CHAPTER VI. USE OF THE WILL. In the practice of the Science of Being Well the will is not used to compel yourself to go when you are not really able to go, or to do things when you are not physically strong enough to do them. You do not direct your will upon your physical body or try to compel the proper performance of internal function by will power. You direct the will upon the mind, and use it in determining what you shall believe, what you shall think, and to what you shall give your attention. The will should never be used upon any person or thing external to you, and it should never be used upon your own body. The sole legitimate use of the will is in determining to what you shall give your attention, and what you shall think about the things to which your attention is given. All belief begins in the will to believe. You cannot always and instantly believe what you will to believe; but you can always will to believe what you want to believe. You want to believe truth about health, and you can will to do so. The statements you have been reading in this book are the truth about health, and you can will to believe them; this must be your first step toward getting well. These are the statements you must will to believe:-- That there is a Thinking Substance from which all things are made, and that man receives the Principle of Health, which is his life, from this Substance. That man himself is Thinking Substance; a mind-body, permeating a physical body, and that as man's thoughts are, so will the functioning of his physical body be. That if man will think only thoughts of perfect health, he must and will cause the internal and involuntary functioning of his body to be the functioning of health, provided that his external and voluntary functioning and attitude are in accordance with his thoughts. When you will to believe these statements, you must also begin to act upon them. You cannot long retain a belief unless you act upon it; you cannot increase a belief until it becomes faith unless you act upon it; and you certainly cannot expect to reap benefits in any way from a belief so long as you act as if the opposite were true. You cannot long have faith in health if you continue to act like a sick person. If you continue to act like a sick person, you cannot help continuing to think of yourself as a sick person; and if you continue to think of yourself as a sick person, you will continue to be a sick person. The first step toward acting externally like a well person is to begin to act internally like a well person. Form your conception of perfect health, and get into the way of thinking about perfect health until it begins to have a definite meaning to you. Picture yourself as doing the things a strong and healthy person would do, and have faith that you can and will do those things in that way; continue this until you have a vivid CONCEPTION of health, and what it means to you. When I speak in this book of a conception of health, I mean a conception that carries with it the idea of the way a healthy person looks and does things. Think of yourself in connection with health until you form a conception of how you would live, appear, act, and do things as a perfectly healthy person. Think about yourself in connection with health until you conceive of yourself, in imagination, as always doing everything in the manner of a well person; until the thought of health conveys the idea of what health means to you. As I have said in a former chapter, you may not be able to form a clear mental image of yourself in perfect health, but you can form a conception of yourself as acting like a healthy person. Form this conception, and then think only thoughts of perfect health in relation to yourself, and, so far as may be possible, in relation to others. When a thought of sickness or disease is presented to you, reject it; do not let it get into your mind; do not entertain or consider it at all. Meet it by thinking health; by thinking that you are well, and by being sincerely grateful for the health you are receiving. Whenever suggestions of disease are coming thick and fast upon you, and you are in a "tight place," fall back upon the exercise of gratitude. Connect yourself with the Supreme; give thanks to God for the perfect health He gives you, and you will soon find yourself able to control your thoughts, and to think what you want to think. In times of doubt, trial, and temptation, the exercise of gratitude is always a sheet anchor which will prevent you from being swept away. Remember that the great essential thing is to SEVER ALL MENTAL RELATIONS WITH DISEASE, AND TO ENTER INTO FULL MENTAL RELATIONSHIP WITH HEALTH. This is the KEY to all mental healing; it is the whole thing. Here we see the secret of the great success of Christian Science; more than any other formulated system of practice, it insists that its converts shall sever relations with disease, and relate themselves fully with health. The healing power of Christian Science is not in its theological formulæ, nor in its denial of matter; but in the fact that it induces the sick to ignore disease as an unreal thing and accept health by faith as a reality. Its failures are made because its practitioners, while thinking in the Certain Way, do not eat, drink, breathe, and sleep in the same way. While there is no healing power in the repetition of strings of words, yet it is a very convenient thing to have the central thoughts so formulated that you can repeat them readily, so that you can use them as affirmations whenever you are surrounded by an environment which gives you adverse suggestions. When those around you begin to talk of sickness and death, close your ears and mentally assert something like the following:-- There is One Substance, and I am that Substance. That Substance is eternal, and it is Life; I am that Substance, and I am Eternal Life. That Substance knows no disease; I am that Substance, and I am Health. Exercise your will power in choosing only those thoughts which are thoughts of health, and arrange your environment so that it shall suggest thoughts of health. Do not have about you books, pictures, or other things which suggest death, disease, deformity, weakness, or age; have only those which convey the ideas of health, power, joy, vitality, and youth. When you are confronted with a book, or anything else which suggests disease, do not give it your attention. Think of your conception of health, and your gratitude, and affirm as above; use your will power to fix your attention upon thoughts of health. In a future chapter I shall touch upon this point again; what I wish to make plain here is that you must think only health, recognize only health, and give your attention only to health; and that you must control thought, recognition, and attention by the use of your will. Do not try to use your will to compel the healthy performance of function within you. The Principle of Health will attend to that, if you give your attention only to thoughts of health. Do not try to exert your will upon the Formless to compel It to give you more vitality or power; it is already placing all the power there is at your service. You do not have to use your will to conquer adverse conditions, or to subdue unfriendly forces; there are no unfriendly forces; there is only One Force, and that force is friendly to you; it is a force which makes for health. Everything in the universe wants you to be well; you have absolutely nothing to overcome but your own habit of thinking in a certain way about disease, and you can do this only by forming a habit of thinking in another Certain Way about health. Man can cause all the internal functions of his body to be performed in a perfectly healthy manner by continuously thinking in a Certain Way, and by performing the external functions in a certain way. He can think in this Certain Way by controlling his attention, and he can control his attention by the use of his will. He can decide what things he will think about.

Summary

In reading this book I hope you have learned the importance of Life Purpose to enabling additional Longevity.

It's really very simple, if we don't have meaning in our lives, then what is the point of living? Our bodies need activity and motivation to stay healthy and strong.

We even provide you some concepts for tools to choose from a variety of alternatives based on various ranking criteria.

Learning this second principle of Personal Longevity lays the basis for you to continue learning and applying the 10 Principles of Personal Longevity to your life.

www.ingramcontent.com/pod-product-compliance
Lightning Source LLC
Chambersburg PA
CBHW051230250726
48655CB00006B/2690